ASD

The Essential Information Guide For Parents Raising A Child With Autism Spectrum Disorder

By

Jenna Everly

TABLE OF CONTENT

INTRODUCTION

Welcome to a journey of understanding and exploration into the diverse and fascinating world of Autism Spectrum Disorder (ASD). This book aims to be your companion—a guide filled with insights, knowledge, and strategies to navigate the intricate landscape of ASD.

Unraveling The Spectrum

Autism Spectrum Disorder is not a single condition; it's a spectrum encompassing a wide range of characteristics, strengths, challenges, and behaviors. Individuals on this spectrum exhibit unique patterns of thought, sensory processing, communication, and social interaction.

Embracing Neurodiversity

In recent years, society has embraced the concept of neurodiversity, recognizing the richness of diverse neurological conditions, including Autism. Embracing neurodiversity means acknowledging and appreciating the unique perspectives and strengths that individuals with Autism bring to the table.

A Holistic Perspective

Understanding Autism extends beyond the individual diagnosed—it encompasses families, caregivers, educators, and society as a whole. This book seeks to provide a holistic view, shedding light on various aspects such as diagnosis, therapies, education, and support systems.

The Journey Ahead

Throughout these pages, we'll explore the nuanced facets of Autism Spectrum Disorder. From decoding the diagnostic criteria to understanding the sensory sensitivities, communication challenges, and interventions, each chapter endeavors to offer clarity and insight.

Bridging Understanding And Compassion

Central to this exploration is fostering empathy and compassion. By delving into the experiences and perspectives of individuals with ASD and those supporting them, we aim to bridge the gap between understanding and genuine compassion.

Empowerment Through Knowledge

Knowledge empowers. Armed with accurate information and strategies, families, educators, therapists, and individuals with ASD can better navigate the challenges and celebrate the unique strengths that come with Autism.

Embracing Hope

Amidst the complexities and uncertainties, there's always hope. Hope for understanding, acceptance, and meaningful inclusion. This book aims to be a beacon of hope, offering insights and tools to facilitate a more inclusive and supportive environment for all.

As we embark on this journey together, let's embrace the richness and diversity that Autism Spectrum Disorder brings to our world. Through knowledge, understanding, and compassion, we can create a more inclusive society where individuals with ASD can thrive and shine.

WHAT IS AUTISM?

Autism, a multifaceted condition known as Autism Spectrum Disorder (ASD), shapes an individual's brain development, affecting behavior, communication, and social interactions uniquely. Described as a spectrum due to its diverse manifestations, it ranges from mild to severe, presenting distinctive challenges and strengths for each person.

Social interaction poses a common challenge for those with autism, encompassing difficulties in interpreting cues, maintaining eye contact, forging relationships, or engaging in conversations. Yet, these challenges vary widely among individuals.

Another facet involves repetitive behaviors or intense interests, such as repetitive movements or fixating on specific subjects. While these behaviors offer comfort, they might appear unusual to others.

Communication hurdles are prevalent, from delayed speech to struggles with non-literal language. Alternative communication methods like visual aids or sign language might be preferred.

Unique talents often emerge, showcasing remarkable abilities in areas like music, art, or memory, termed "special interests," adding joy and fulfillment.

The cause remains complex, possibly involving genetic and environmental factors. Ongoing research seeks deeper insights into autism's origins and better ways to support affected individuals.

Diagnosis involves observing behaviors and developmental milestones, utilizing standardized tests by healthcare professionals. Early intervention is pivotal for optimal support.

Support strategies, including tailored therapies and educational interventions, aim to address individual needs. Community resources and support groups are invaluable for both individuals with autism and their families.

Fostering an inclusive environment that embraces neurodiversity is crucial, promoting understanding and appreciation for the unique strengths of those with autism.

Autism is not a condition to be "cured"; it's an intrinsic aspect of an individual's identity. With understanding, support, and opportunities, those with autism can lead fulfilling lives and contribute meaningfully to society.

SIGNS AND SYMPTOMS OF AUTISM

Recognizing the signs and symptoms of autism is essential for early identification and support. Autism Spectrum Disorder (ASD) manifests in various ways, and being aware of the key indicators can aid in understanding and seeking appropriate assistance for individuals.

One of the primary signs of autism is difficulty in social interaction. Children with autism might show reduced interest in socializing or playing with others. They might not respond to their name being called, struggle to make eye contact, or have difficulty understanding gestures and facial expressions. Some children may prefer to play alone and find it challenging to engage in reciprocal conversations or make friends.

Another noticeable aspect involves communication challenges. Children with autism might exhibit delayed speech development or have difficulty initiating or maintaining conversations. Some may repeat words or phrases (echolalia) without understanding their meanings. Others might have a vast vocabulary but struggle with using language in social contexts or understanding non-literal language like jokes or sarcasm.

Repetitive behaviors and a need for routine are also common in individuals with autism. Children might engage in repetitive movements like hand-flapping, rocking, or spinning objects. They might insist on following specific routines and become upset if there's a change. Some children with autism develop intense interests in specific topics, objects, or activities, focusing extensively on them.

Sensory sensitivities are prevalent among individuals with autism. They might be oversensitive or under sensitive to sensory stimuli like light, sound, touch, taste, or smell. For instance, they might cover their ears in response to loud noises or become distressed in bright lighting.

It's important to remember that while these signs and symptoms are common in autism, not every individual will display all of them. The severity and combination of symptoms vary widely among individuals on the spectrum.

Recognizing these signs early on is crucial. Parents and caregivers are often the first to notice differences in their child's development. If there's a concern, seeking evaluation by healthcare professionals, such as pediatricians, psychologists, or developmental specialists, can lead to early diagnosis and intervention.

Early intervention services can play a significant role in supporting children with autism. These services might include speech therapy, occupational therapy, behavioral therapy, and educational interventions tailored to the child's specific needs and strengths.

It's important to note that while the signs of autism usually appear in early childhood, some individuals might not receive a diagnosis until later in life. This could be due to various factors, including milder symptoms that were overlooked or other coexisting conditions that masked the signs of autism.

Understanding and recognizing the signs and symptoms of autism create pathways for timely intervention and support. It's crucial to approach each individual with empathy and understanding, recognizing their unique strengths and challenges. By fostering an inclusive environment and providing appropriate resources, we can ensure that individuals with autism receive the support they need to thrive.

One common question many parents and caregivers have is: At what age can autism be diagnosed?

EARLY SIGNS AND DIAGNOSIS

The signs of autism can emerge as early as 18 months, though some children might not display noticeable symptoms until they are older. Typically, a formal diagnosis can occur around the ages of 2 to 3 years old. Nevertheless, it's crucial to emphasize that autism holds the potential for diagnosis across various stages of life, irrespective of age.

Diagnosis Process

The diagnosis of autism involves comprehensive assessments by healthcare professionals, such as pediatricians, psychologists, or developmental specialists. They use specific criteria outlined in the Diagnostic and Statistical Manual of Mental Disorders (DSM-5) to evaluate a child's behavior, communication skills, and social interactions.

Early Indicators

Certain behaviors and developmental milestones might indicate the possibility of autism in children. These indicators can include:

Social Communication Differences: Difficulty making eye contact, not responding to their name, or having challenges with sharing emotions or interests with others.

Language Delay or Regression: Some children might not develop language skills on par with their peers or may lose previously acquired language abilities.

Repetitive Behaviors: Engaging in repetitive movements like hand-flapping, rocking, or having rigid adherence to routines.
Importance of Early Detection

The timely identification and proactive support play a pivotal role in assisting children diagnosed with autism spectrum disorder. Identifying ASD early allows for timely access to specialized services and therapies that can significantly improve the child's development and quality of life. These interventions may include speech therapy, occupational therapy, behavioral therapy, and educational support tailored to the child's needs.

Challenges In Diagnosis

While some children display clear signs of autism early on, others might present with subtler symptoms or have co-occurring conditions, making the diagnosis more challenging. Additionally, cultural differences, limited access to healthcare, and varying levels of awareness about autism can also impact the timing of diagnosis.

Diagnostic Tools And Assessments

Healthcare professionals use various tools and assessments to diagnose autism. These assessments involve observing the child's behavior and interactions, interviewing parents or caregivers about the child's development, and sometimes conducting standardized tests to evaluate specific skills.

Continuum Of Development

Autism's nature as a spectrum disorder signifies its diverse presentation in every person it affects, leading to unique manifestations and experiences for each individual. The severity of symptoms can range from mild to severe, and the developmental trajectory varies widely. As a result, there is no one-size-fits-all approach to diagnosing autism.

Late Diagnosis

In some cases, individuals might receive an autism diagnosis later in life, even as teenagers or adults. This can happen due to various reasons, including masking or camouflaging behaviors to fit in socially, or when symptoms become more noticeable or disruptive as they age.

The age at which autism is diagnosed can vary significantly from child to child. Early identification and intervention remain pivotal, but diagnosis at any age allows individuals and their families to access the support and resources needed for optimal development and improved quality of life.

Remember, every child is unique, and seeking professional guidance if you suspect autism is crucial for early detection and appropriate support.

IS THERE A CURE FOR AUTISM?

As of now, there isn't a singular cure for autism. Autism is considered a spectrum disorder because it presents differently in each individual. Some people with autism may have mild symptoms, while others may face more significant challenges. Since autism is complex and varies greatly among individuals, finding a single cure that works universally for everyone hasn't been achieved yet.

However, it's essential to highlight that various therapies and interventions are available to help individuals manage and improve symptoms associated with autism. These interventions aim to enhance communication skills, social interaction, and behavioral patterns. Early intervention programs, such as Applied Behavior

Analysis (ABA), speech therapy, occupational therapy, and social skills training, have shown positive results in improving the lives of individuals with autism.

Medication is another aspect of managing certain symptoms associated with autism. Some medications can help manage behavioral challenges, anxiety, depression, or attention issues that might accompany autism. However, these medications are aimed at alleviating specific symptoms and don't constitute a cure for autism itself.

It's crucial to understand that autism is not a disease that can be eradicated. Rather, it's a neurological difference that shapes an individual's perception, behavior, and interaction with the world. Many people with autism lead fulfilling lives, contribute to society, and excel in various fields.

Research in the field of autism is ongoing. Scientists and researchers are continually investigating the causes of autism and exploring potential treatments or interventions that could further help individuals on the spectrum. However, finding a definitive cure remains a complex challenge due to the multifaceted nature of autism.

The focus within the scientific community is gradually shifting towards acceptance and support rather than seeking a cure. Instead of aiming to change individuals with autism, efforts are directed towards providing them with the necessary tools, support, and understanding to thrive in society.

It's crucial to embrace neurodiversity, recognizing and valuing the differences in how individuals think, learn, and interact with the world. Acceptance and support foster a more inclusive society where individuals with autism can reach their full potential without feeling pressured to conform to neurotypical standards.

WHAT CAUSES AUTISM?

Understanding the causes of autism is an ongoing area of research with multiple factors believed to contribute to its development.

Genetics:

Autism's development is substantially influenced by genetic elements. Research suggests that certain genetic mutations or variations can increase the likelihood of ASD. These genetic changes might be inherited from parents or occur spontaneously. Nevertheless, it's crucial to acknowledge that not every person carrying these genetic variations will necessarily manifest autism.

Environmental Factors:

Environmental influences during pregnancy and early infancy may also contribute to the development of autism. Factors such as exposure to certain chemicals, infections, or complications during pregnancy might play a role in increasing the risk of ASD. Yet, researchers continue their exploration into identifying the precise environmental catalysts involved in this phenomenon.

Brain Development:
Alterations in brain development are thought to be linked to the development of autism. Early brain overgrowth or differences in the structure and connectivity of the brain in individuals with ASD have been observed. These differences might affect how the brain processes information and how individuals with autism perceive and interact with the world around them.

Neurological Differences:
Individuals with autism often exhibit neurological differences in how their brains function. These differences might affect sensory processing, social interactions, communication, and repetitive behaviors characteristic of ASD. Researchers are exploring these neurological variations to better understand their role in autism.

Potential Risk Factors:

Certain factors might increase the risk of autism but don't directly cause it. These include advanced parental age at the time of conception, premature birth, low birth weight, and maternal illnesses during pregnancy. While these factors might slightly elevate the risk, they alone do not cause autism.

No Single Cause:

It's important to emphasize that there is no single known cause of autism. Rather, it's believed to be a complex interplay of genetic, environmental, and neurological factors. Each individual with autism is unique, and the combination of factors contributing to their condition can vary significantly.

DIAGNOSIS AND SUPPORT

Diagnosing autism involves observing behavioral patterns and developmental milestones. Swift detection in the early stages remains pivotal for accessing tailored interventions and essential support services. While there is no cure for autism, various interventions, therapies, and support networks can help individuals with ASD lead fulfilling lives and reach their full potential.

HOW DOES AUTISM AFFECT LEARNING AND DEVELOPMENT?

SENSORY SENSITIVITIES

For individuals with ASD, sensory sensitivities can significantly affect their learning. Certain sounds, lights, textures, or even smells might cause distress or discomfort, making it harder to concentrate in a traditional classroom environment.

Sensory sensitivities are a crucial aspect to consider for individuals with Autism Spectrum Disorder (ASD). These sensitivities can make everyday experiences overwhelming. Imagine being hypersensitive to common things like noises, bright lights, specific textures, or certain smells. For someone with ASD, these stimuli might not just be a minor annoyance but could cause extreme discomfort or distress, making it tough to focus or engage in a typical classroom setting.

In a classroom, the flickering of fluorescent lights, the hum of electronics, or the scratchy texture of certain materials can be incredibly distracting or even painful for someone with sensory sensitivities. For instance, what might seem like a faint background noise to most people could be unbearable for someone with hypersensitivity to sound.

Understanding these sensitivities is key to creating an environment that supports learning for individuals with ASD. By making small adjustments like using softer lighting, providing noise-canceling headphones, offering alternative textures for materials, or even using gentle scents or removing strong odors, educators can create a more comfortable and inclusive space that helps these individuals focus and thrive in their learning journey.

DIFFICULTY WITH SOCIAL INTERACTIONS

Autism Spectrum Disorder (ASD) often affects social interaction, posing challenges in learning and daily life. Individuals with ASD might struggle with understanding social cues, body language, facial expressions, and tone of voice. This difficulty can hinder their ability to form relationships, engage in conversations, or comprehend social nuances.

Moreover, those with ASD might find it challenging to initiate or sustain conversations, leading to isolation or difficulty in group settings. This impacts their learning as social interaction plays a pivotal role in educational environments. Classroom discussions, group projects, and cooperative learning settings may pose challenges for individuals with ASD due to these difficulties.

Furthermore, the struggle to interpret non-verbal communication can affect their learning in various subjects. For instance, in subjects involving interpreting emotions or understanding implicit social cues (such as literature or history), individuals with ASD might face hurdles comprehending the underlying context.

To address these challenges, various strategies are employed, including social skills training, communication therapies, and creating structured environments that accommodate individual needs. Implementing specialized teaching methods tailored to the unique learning styles of individuals with ASD can significantly support their educational journey.

Overall, the difficulties in social interaction experienced by individuals with autism can significantly impact their learning process, emphasizing the importance of tailored support and understanding in educational settings.

REPETITIVE BEHAVIORS AND ROUTINES

Repetitive behaviors and adherence to routines are often key characteristics in individuals with autism that can significantly impact their learning experiences. These behaviors, often termed "restricted and repetitive behaviors" (RRBs), manifest in various forms such as repetitive movements (like hand flapping or rocking), insistence on sameness, strict adherence to specific routines or rituals, and an intense focus on particular interests.

In the realm of learning, these behaviors might present challenges by interfering with the flexibility required to adapt to new situations or learning methods. For instance, a strong preference for routine can make it difficult to transition between tasks or accept changes in schedules, potentially disrupting the learning process. Additionally, an intense focus on specific topics or interests might lead to difficulties in engaging with a broader curriculum or interacting with peers who have different interests.

Educational strategies tailored to accommodate these behaviors are crucial. Providing predictability through consistent schedules and clear communication about changes can help mitigate anxiety and resistance to alterations in routine. Incorporating the individual's specific interests into learning activities can enhance engagement and motivation. Breaking down tasks into smaller, structured steps can also facilitate learning and reduce feelings of overwhelm.

Recognizing and understanding these behaviors is pivotal in creating inclusive learning environments that cater to the diverse needs of individuals with autism. Empathy, patience, and tailored support can empower these individuals to navigate the learning process more effectively, leveraging their unique strengths and abilities.

ARE THERE SPECIFIC THERAPIES OR TREATMENTS FOR AUTISM?

Autism spectrum disorder (ASD) is a neurodevelopmental condition that affects individuals differently. Because of this diversity, there isn't a one-size-fits-all approach to therapy or treatment. Instead, a range of interventions and therapies are available to help manage symptoms and support individuals with autism in various aspects of their lives.

1. Behavioral Therapies:

Behavioral therapies are among the most common and effective treatments for autism. Applied Behavior Analysis (ABA) is one such therapy that focuses on improving specific behaviors. It uses positive reinforcement to encourage desired behaviors and reduce unwanted ones. ABA can be tailored to address communication, social skills, academics, and daily living skills.

Behavioral therapies are widely used in treating autism spectrum disorder (ASD) due to their focus on improving specific behaviors, communication skills, and social interactions. Applied Behavior Analysis (ABA) is one of the most common and extensively researched behavioral therapies for individuals with autism. ABA aims to increase desirable behaviors and decrease harmful or challenging ones by breaking down tasks into smaller, manageable steps and using positive reinforcement techniques.

Another effective approach is Pivotal Response Treatment (PRT), which focuses on pivotal areas like motivation, responding to multiple cues, self-management, and initiating social interactions. PRT aims to improve motivation and self-initiation while targeting various behaviors in naturalistic settings.

Moreover, Social Skills Training helps individuals with autism learn and practice appropriate social behaviors, including communication, understanding social cues, and engaging in conversations or play activities.

Early Start Denver Model (ESDM) is another comprehensive intervention designed for young children with autism. It combines ABA techniques with developmental and relationship-based approaches to improve social communication, cognitive, and adaptive behaviors.

Overall, these behavioral therapies provide structured, individualized interventions aimed at enhancing communication, social skills, and behavior management in individuals with autism, helping them lead more fulfilling lives.

2. Occupational Therapy:

Occupational therapy (OT) for autism focuses on enhancing an individual's ability to engage in daily activities, improve social interactions, and develop essential life skills. This therapy aims to address sensory, motor, and cognitive challenges that individuals with autism may face.

OT professionals use tailored interventions to help individuals with autism manage sensory sensitivities, improve motor skills, regulate emotions, and enhance social participation. They employ various activities like sensory integration techniques, play-based exercises, and structured routines to promote independence and functional abilities.

Sensory integration techniques assist in managing sensory sensitivities commonly experienced by those with autism, helping them regulate responses to sensory stimuli. Play-based activities aid in developing fine and gross motor skills, while structured routines foster predictability and organization, supporting individuals in managing daily tasks effectively.

Moreover, occupational therapists collaborate closely with families, educators, and other healthcare professionals to create individualized treatment plans that address specific needs and goals. By offering a holistic approach, occupational therapy helps individuals with autism lead fulfilling lives by maximizing their potential and fostering independence in various aspects of daily living.

3. Speech Therapy:

Speech therapy is a critical part of autism treatment, focusing on improving communication skills. It helps individuals with autism spectrum disorder (ASD) enhance their ability to understand and use language, gestures, and social cues.

Therapists use various techniques tailored to each person's needs. For nonverbal individuals, they might introduce alternative communication methods like sign language or picture boards. For those with limited speech, therapists work on expanding vocabulary, sentence structure, and articulation.

Additionally, speech therapy targets social communication, teaching how to initiate and maintain conversations, interpret nonverbal cues, and comprehend figurative language.

The goal is to improve overall communication skills, fostering better interaction, social integration, and independence for individuals with autism. Each therapy plan is personalized, adapting to the unique strengths and challenges of the person undergoing treatment.

4. Social Skills Training:

Social skills training is an essential component of autism therapy, focusing on enhancing interpersonal interactions and social understanding. It helps individuals with autism spectrum disorder (ASD) navigate social situations more effectively.

The training typically involves various techniques tailored to the individual's needs. Therapists use role-playing, modeling, and direct instruction to teach social cues, body language, and appropriate social behaviors.

Key areas addressed in social skills training include:

Understanding Social Cues: Teaching individuals to recognize facial expressions, tone of voice, and body language to understand others' emotions and intentions.

Initiating and Maintaining Conversations: Helping individuals start conversations, take turns speaking, and stay on topic during interactions.

Developing Empathy and Perspective-Taking: Encouraging individuals to understand others' feelings, viewpoints, and experiences.

Problem-Solving and Conflict Resolution: Teaching strategies to handle conflicts, cope with social challenges, and navigate difficult situations.

Group Interaction Skills: Engaging in group activities to foster teamwork, sharing, and cooperation.

Therapists customize programs based on the individual's strengths and challenges, gradually building skills through practice, feedback, and reinforcement. Consistent practice in real-life situations helps generalize these skills beyond therapy sessions, promoting better social integration and relationships for individuals with autism.

5. Sensory Integration Therapy:

Sensory Integration Therapy is a method used to assist individuals, particularly those with autism, in processing and responding to sensory information. It aims to help people better manage sensory input from their environment. The therapy involves activities and exercises that stimulate the senses, such as touch, smell, sight, sound, and movement, to assist individuals in regulating their responses to sensory input.

During Sensory Integration Therapy, a trained therapist designs activities that provide controlled sensory input, gradually helping individuals become more accustomed to and better able to manage different sensory experiences. For instance, this might include activities like swinging, bouncing, brushing the skin, or playing with various textures to help desensitize or heighten sensory responses based on the individual's needs.

The goal of this therapy is to improve an individual's ability to process and respond to sensory information effectively, which can lead to better attention, communication, behavior, and overall functioning.

It's essential to note that while some evidence supports the benefits of Sensory Integration Therapy, its effectiveness varies from person to person. The therapy is often part of a comprehensive treatment plan tailored to the specific needs of the individual with autism.

6. Medication:

While medication doesn't treat autism itself, it can manage certain associated symptoms like anxiety, depression, hyperactivity, or aggression. Medication should be prescribed and monitored by healthcare professionals.

7. Alternative Therapies:

Alternative therapies for autism encompass a range of approaches beyond conventional medicine. While these methods vary widely and often lack robust scientific validation, they're often sought out by individuals seeking complementary or alternative options for managing autism spectrum disorder (ASD).

Dietary Interventions: Some alternative therapies involve dietary changes, such as gluten-free or casein-free diets, as some believe that certain foods exacerbate symptoms of ASD. However, scientific evidence supporting these dietary interventions is limited.

Nutritional Supplements: Some families explore the use of supplements like vitamins, minerals, or other compounds, such as omega-3 fatty acids or probiotics, believing they might alleviate some symptoms. Yet, conclusive evidence supporting their efficacy is insufficient.

Mind-Body Practices: Yoga, meditation, and acupuncture are among the mind-body practices that some individuals explore for managing stress and anxiety associated with ASD. However, scientific evidence on their effectiveness specifically for autism is inconclusive.

It's important to note that while some individuals and families report positive experiences with alternative therapies, scientific evidence validating their effectiveness for treating core symptoms of ASD is often limited or conflicting. Before pursuing any alternative therapy, consulting with healthcare professionals, including physicians and autism specialists, is crucial to ensure safety and appropriate guidance.

Additionally, a holistic approach that combines evidence-based interventions with alternative therapies, if desired, might be the most comprehensive way to address the diverse needs of individuals with ASD.

8. Parent-Mediated Therapies:

Parent-mediated therapy in the context of autism treatment involves empowering parents or caregivers to actively participate in and deliver interventions tailored to their child's needs. This approach acknowledges the vital role parents play in their child's development and focuses on equipping them with strategies to support and promote their child's communication, social interaction, and overall well-being.

Early Start Denver Model (ESDM): This evidence-based intervention utilizes parent-mediated strategies within a comprehensive curriculum designed for children with autism aged 12 to 48 months. It emphasizes naturalistic learning opportunities embedded in everyday activities and interactions to enhance social communication skills.

Pivotal Response Treatment (PRT): PRT involves teaching parents techniques based on principles of applied behavior analysis (ABA) to improve pivotal behaviors, such as motivation, initiations, self-management, and responding to multiple cues. Parents learn to create environments that encourage their child's social communication.

Responsive Teaching: This approach focuses on enhancing parents' responsiveness to their child's cues, interests, and communication attempts. It involves teaching parents how to recognize and respond effectively to their child's communication attempts, thereby promoting language and social development.

Communication-Based Interventions:
Parents are taught specific communication strategies, such as using visual supports, augmentative and alternative communication (AAC) devices, or implementing specific techniques like the Picture Exchange Communication System (PECS) at home to facilitate their child's communication skills.

Social Skills Training for Parents: Training programs help parents understand social skills deficits in autism and teach them strategies to promote social interactions, perspective-taking, and friendship skills within various contexts, including home and community settings.

Tailored Support and Education: Professionals provide individualized guidance and education to parents, considering their child's unique needs and challenges. This might involve ongoing coaching, workshops, or resources that empower parents to implement effective strategies.

Parent-mediated therapy recognizes the significance of the parent-child relationship and the potential impact parents can have on their child's development. It not only aims to enhance the child's skills but also supports and educates parents, empowering them to effectively engage with their child in daily activities to foster growth and development.

It's important for parents considering this approach to work closely with trained professionals, such as speech therapists, behavior analysts, or developmental specialists, to ensure they receive appropriate guidance, support, and resources to implement these interventions effectively and suitably for their child's needs.

9. Technology-Based Interventions:

There's a growing use of technology-based interventions, such as apps and virtual reality programs, to aid in skill development, communication, and behavior management for individuals with autism.

Technology-based interventions in the realm of autism treatment encompass a wide array of tools and applications designed to assist individuals with autism spectrum disorder (ASD) in various aspects of their lives. These interventions leverage technological advancements to enhance communication, social skills, learning, and daily functioning for individuals on the spectrum.

Communication Aids and Apps: Numerous apps and software cater to augmentative and alternative communication (AAC) needs. These tools facilitate communication by using pictures, symbols, text-to-speech functionalities, and customizable interfaces to help individuals with limited verbal abilities express themselves effectively.

Social Skills Training Apps: Technology offers interactive programs and apps designed explicitly for teaching and practicing social skills. These tools provide visual aids, scenarios, and interactive activities to help individuals with ASD learn social cues, conversation techniques, and appropriate social behaviors.

Educational Software: Tailored educational software and apps address diverse learning styles and needs. They cover a range of subjects, offering interactive lessons, adaptive learning environments, and engaging activities to support academic development and cognitive skills.

Virtual Reality (Vr) And Augmented Reality (Ar):
VR and AR technologies are increasingly utilized to create simulated environments for individuals with ASD. These immersive experiences help in social skills training, sensory integration, and real-world scenario practice in a controlled and supportive setting.

Wearable Devices: Some wearable devices, such as smartwatches or specialized gadgets, provide prompts, reminders, or cues for individuals with ASD to manage their daily routines, transitions, and activities more independently.

Sensor-Based Technologies: These tools use sensors or trackers to monitor and manage sensory sensitivities, sleep patterns, or behavioral patterns. They can offer insights into triggers for meltdowns or stressors, aiding caregivers in developing strategies to mitigate them.

Robot-Assisted Therapies: Robotics, including humanoid robots or specialized devices, are utilized in therapeutic settings to engage individuals with ASD in structured interactions, prompting social engagement, communication, and emotional expression.

While technology-based interventions offer promising avenues for supporting individuals with ASD, it's essential to approach their use with careful consideration:

Individualization: Interventions should be tailored to the specific needs and preferences of the individual with ASD.

Professional Guidance: Consulting therapists, educators, or specialists is crucial to ensure the selected technology aligns with therapeutic goals and suits the individual's requirements.

Monitoring and Assessment: Regular monitoring and evaluation of the technology's effectiveness in meeting the intended goals are essential for ongoing adjustments and improvements.

Integrating technology-based interventions into a comprehensive treatment plan alongside other evidence-based therapies can enhance the overall support and development of individuals with ASD.

10. Early Intervention Programs:

The Early Intervention Program (EIP) dedicated to autism spectrum disorder (ASD) pioneers a structured strategy pinpointing and tackling developmental hurdles in children diagnosed with ASD. This specialized initiative commences upon the emergence of autism-related signs, often before age three, recognizing the pivotal role of early intervention in fostering superior outcomes.

Within EIP lies a spectrum of personalized therapies and interventions, such as Applied Behavior Analysis (ABA), speech therapy, occupational therapy, social skills training, and sensory integration therapy. Its principal objective revolves around amplifying communication proficiencies, refining social interactions, managing behavior, and bolstering everyday life skills.

This comprehensive program thrives on a collaborative multidisciplinary team, inclusive of therapists, psychologists, educators, and engaged parents. A cornerstone of success involves family integration, empowering parents with tailored strategies to nurture their child's development within their home environment.

Studies affirm the significant impact of early intervention in augmenting the trajectory of children with autism, potentially mitigating symptom severity and heightening their adaptability across diverse settings.

It's crucial to acknowledge that EIP's efficacy hinges on diverse factors including individual needs, intervention consistency, and program quality. Timely identification and initiation of customized interventions remain paramount in realizing the potential of children with autism spectrum disorder.

It's important to note that what works for one individual with autism might not be as effective for another. A combination of therapies tailored to the individual's needs, strengths, and challenges tends to yield the best results.

Before starting any therapy or treatment, consulting with healthcare professionals, such as pediatricians, psychologists, or developmental specialists, is vital. They can help determine the most suitable interventions based on the individual's specific needs.

WHAT ARE SOME COMMON MISCONCEPTIONS ABOUT AUTISM?

There are several common misconceptions about Autism Spectrum Disorder (ASD) that often lead to misunderstanding and misinformation. Let's explore and debunk some of these misconceptions.

Misconception 1: Autism Is A Singular, Uniform Condition

One of the most prevalent misconceptions about autism is that it presents itself in a standardized way. In reality, autism is a spectrum disorder, meaning it encompasses a wide range of characteristics, behaviors, and challenges. Each person with autism is unique, with their own strengths, abilities, and areas where they may need support.

Misconception 2: People With Autism Lack Empathy Or Emotions

Contrary to this belief, individuals with autism do experience emotions and empathy. However, they might express and interpret these feelings in different ways compared to neurotypical individuals. Difficulty in understanding social cues or nonverbal communication does not equate to a lack of empathy.

Misconception 3: Autism Is Caused By Vaccines

Countless scientific investigations have refuted this misunderstanding, demonstrating no established correlation between vaccines and the onset of autism. Extensive research has consistently shown that vaccines are safe and do not cause autism.

Misconception 4: Individuals With Autism Are All Geniuses Or Have Extraordinary Skills

While some individuals with autism possess exceptional skills or talents in specific areas like mathematics, music, or art, this is not a universal characteristic. The spectrum encompasses a wide range of abilities, and not everyone with autism possesses savant-like abilities.

Misconception 5: Autism Is A Childhood Disorder That Disappears With Age

Autism is a lifelong condition. While early interventions and therapies can significantly help individuals with autism develop essential skills, the core traits and characteristics of autism persist throughout their lives. With appropriate support, individuals with autism can continue to learn and grow, adapting to different life stages.

Misconception 6: Individuals With Autism Don't Want Social Interaction

While some individuals with autism might experience challenges in social situations, many desire social interaction and connections. Difficulty with social communication doesn't necessarily mean they don't want friendships or relationships; rather, they might require support and alternative means of communication.

Misconception 7: Autism Only Affects Boys

Historically, autism was thought to predominantly affect boys. However, we now understand that autism occurs in all genders. Diagnosis might have been biased in the past, leading to an underrepresentation of girls and non-binary individuals on the spectrum.

Misconception 8: Individuals With Autism Can't Lead Independent Lives

This misconception overlooks the fact that many individuals with autism can live independently with appropriate support. While some may require assistance or accommodations, with the right resources and guidance, many individuals with autism can achieve varying degrees of independence and lead fulfilling lives.

Misconception 9: All Individuals With Autism Have Intellectual Disabilities

Autism and intellectual disability are distinct conditions. While some individuals with autism might have intellectual disabilities, many others have average or above-average intelligence. It's important not to assume intellectual abilities based solely on an autism diagnosis.

Misconception 10: Autism Can Be "Cured"
Autism is not a disease or something that needs curing. Rather, it's a neurological difference. Early interventions and therapies can help individuals with autism develop skills and cope with challenges, but there is no "cure" for autism because it's an inherent part of a person's identity.

Understanding and addressing these misconceptions are crucial in creating a more inclusive and supportive environment for individuals with autism. Embracing neurodiversity and acknowledging the strengths and unique qualities of individuals on the spectrum can pave the way for greater acceptance and inclusion in our society.

HOW DOES AUTISM DIFFER IN GIRLS AND BOYS?

Autism Spectrum Disorder (ASD) affects individuals in various ways, but the differences between how it manifests in girls and boys often pose an interesting perspective.

Firstly, diagnosing ASD in girls can sometimes be trickier compared to boys. Girls might display different signs or mask their symptoms more effectively, making it harder for professionals to identify ASD early on. Boys, on the other hand, often exhibit more noticeable symptoms, like repetitive behaviors or intense focus on specific topics, which can lead to earlier recognition.

When it comes to social interactions, girls with ASD might appear more socially adept on the surface compared to boys. They might mimic behaviors of their peers, making it less obvious that they struggle with social cues. Boys with ASD tend to stand out more due to challenges in maintaining eye contact, sharing interests, or engaging in reciprocal conversations.

Communication patterns also differ between genders. Girls might use more sophisticated language and have a larger vocabulary than boys with ASD, which can sometimes camouflage their difficulties in communication. Boys might exhibit more literal interpretations of language and face challenges in understanding sarcasm or figures of speech.

Sensory sensitivities, a common aspect of ASD, can be distinct between genders. Girls might cope better or have a higher tolerance for sensory stimuli, making it less noticeable that they experience sensory overload. Boys might display more overt reactions to sensory inputs, like covering their ears in response to loud noises or being sensitive to certain textures.

Another aspect to consider is special interests or obsessions. Boys with ASD might intensely focus on objects or specific subjects, displaying their interests openly and noticeably. In contrast, girls might have more socially acceptable interests, making it less apparent that their fixation is linked to ASD.

Understanding these differences between how ASD manifests in girls and boys is crucial for early identification and tailored support. It's important to remember that ASD doesn't manifest uniformly and can vary widely within each individual, regardless of gender. Awareness of these differences helps professionals and caregivers provide more nuanced and effective support for individuals with ASD.

Recognizing and appreciating the diversity within ASD allows for a more inclusive and understanding approach. Creating an environment that accommodates these differences helps individuals on the spectrum thrive, regardless of their gender.

WHAT ARE SOME CO-OCCURING CONDITIONS WITH AUTISM?

Discussing co-occurring conditions with Autism Spectrum Disorder (ASD) is essential. It's common for individuals diagnosed with ASD to also experience other conditions simultaneously. Understanding these co-occurring conditions is crucial for effective management and support.

One frequent co-occurring condition is Attention-Deficit/Hyperactivity Disorder (ADHD). Both ASD and ADHD share certain symptoms, like difficulty focusing and impulsivity. However, individuals with ASD might have more trouble with social interaction, while those with ADHD might struggle more with hyperactivity.

Anxiety disorders are also commonly seen alongside ASD. Children and adults with ASD might feel overwhelmed or anxious in social situations, leading to avoidance or distress. It's vital to recognize these signs and offer appropriate support.

Depression can also co-occur with ASD. Challenges in social interactions, difficulty in communication, or coping with sensory sensitivities may contribute to feelings of isolation or sadness, leading to depression.

Another co-occurring condition is Epilepsy. Research shows a higher prevalence of epilepsy among individuals with ASD. Seizures can impact behavior and cognitive abilities, making it crucial to manage both conditions concurrently.

Sensory processing difficulties are prevalent among individuals with ASD. This condition involves challenges in processing sensory information, leading to over or under-sensitivity to sights, sounds, touch, taste, or smells. These difficulties can affect daily functioning and might lead to distress or discomfort.

Gastrointestinal (GI) issues are also observed in some individuals with ASD. While the connection isn't fully understood, studies suggest a higher prevalence of GI symptoms like constipation, diarrhea, or abdominal pain in those with ASD.

Intellectual disabilities can co-occur with ASD, although not in every case. Some individuals with ASD might have intellectual disabilities, impacting their cognitive abilities and learning.

Moreover, conditions like Obsessive-Compulsive Disorder (OCD) or Tourette Syndrome can also co-occur with ASD, though not as frequently as the previously mentioned conditions.

Understanding these co-occurring conditions is crucial for families, caregivers, and professionals working with individuals on the autism spectrum. Early identification and tailored interventions can significantly improve the quality of life for those facing these challenges.

Each person with ASD is unique, and the manifestation of these co-occurring conditions can vary widely. Therefore, a personalized approach to intervention and support is vital. Collaborating with healthcare professionals, therapists, educators, and support groups can provide a holistic approach to address these co-occurring conditions effectively.

Remember, the presence of co-occurring conditions doesn't diminish an individual's strengths or potential. With the right support and understanding, individuals with ASD can thrive and lead fulfilling lives, contributing their unique perspectives and talents to the world around them.

HOW DOES AUTISM CHANGE WITH AGE?

Autism, like many developmental conditions, can evolve and change over time as individuals grow older. Understanding how Autism changes with age is crucial for families, caregivers, and professionals involved in supporting individuals on the spectrum.

Early Childhood (Ages 2-5):
In early childhood, signs of Autism Spectrum Disorder (ASD) often become noticeable. Children might exhibit delayed speech, difficulty in social interactions, repetitive behaviors, or sensory sensitivities. Early intervention during this phase, such as speech therapy or behavioral interventions, can make a significant difference in a child's development.

Middle Childhood (Ages 6-12):
During these years, children with ASD might experience improvements in certain areas. With appropriate support and interventions, they

might develop better communication skills, learn coping strategies for sensory sensitivities, and show progress in social interactions. However, challenges might persist in areas like socializing or adapting to new situations.

Adolescence (Ages 13-18):
Adolescence often brings new challenges for individuals with ASD. Hormonal changes, increased social expectations, and transitioning to more complex social environments, like high school, can be overwhelming. Some may face difficulties in understanding social cues or managing emotions. Others might develop special interests or skills they can leverage positively.

Adulthood (Ages 18 and beyond):
As individuals transition into adulthood, some aspects of ASD might become less prominent, while others persist. With continued support, many individuals with ASD can lead independent and fulfilling lives. However, challenges in social situations, finding

employment, or managing daily routines might still exist. Some might discover strengths in certain fields due to their unique perspectives and abilities.

Changes in Behaviors and Traits:
It's important to note that certain behaviors associated with ASD might change over time. For instance, some individuals might become more adept at social interactions, while others might continue to struggle. Special interests can also evolve or intensify, leading to new skills or opportunities for growth.

Mental Health and Co-Occurring Conditions:
Throughout life, individuals with ASD might encounter mental health challenges such as anxiety, depression, or ADHD. As they age, these co-occurring conditions might become more pronounced, requiring tailored interventions and support.

Adapting to Transitions:
Transitions, such as moving from one educational level to another, entering the workforce, or living independently, can be particularly challenging for individuals with ASD. Providing structured support during these transitions is crucial to help them navigate changes successfully.

Individualized Support and Understanding:
Understanding that Autism changes differently for each individual is key. Some might experience significant progress in certain areas, while others might require ongoing support. Approaching each person with empathy,

patience, and individualized interventions can significantly enhance their quality of life.

Community Involvement and Acceptance:
Creating inclusive communities that value and embrace neurodiversity is essential. By fostering acceptance and understanding, we can create environments that support individuals with ASD as they navigate different stages of life.

Autism is a lifelong developmental condition that changes and evolves with time. Early intervention, continued support, and a deeper understanding of individual needs can greatly enhance the lives of those on the autism spectrum as they journey through different stages of life.

WHAT ARE THE STRENGTHS ASSOCIATED WITH ASD?

Autism Spectrum Disorder (ASD) is often associated with a range of strengths and unique abilities. Some of these include:

Exceptional Focus: Individuals with ASD often exhibit intense focus and attention to detail in areas of interest. This focused attention can lead to expertise in specific subjects or skills.

Pattern Recognition: Many individuals with ASD excel in recognizing and understanding patterns, whether in numbers, music, or visual elements. This skill often translates into strengths in fields like mathematics, music, coding, or art.

Creativity: ASD is often linked to heightened creativity and original thinking. Some individuals demonstrate innovative problem-solving abilities and unique ways of approaching challenges.

Memory: Some individuals with ASD possess impressive memory skills, especially related to factual information or areas of personal interest. This can be advantageous in certain academic or professional settings.

Honesty and Integrity: Individuals with ASD are often known for their sincerity and honesty. Their straightforwardness can be an asset in relationships and interactions.

Dedication and Commitment: When engaged in activities or projects of interest, individuals with ASD tend to demonstrate high levels of dedication and persistence, leading to accomplishments in their chosen fields.

Specialized Knowledge: Many individuals with ASD develop deep and detailed knowledge in specific subjects due to their focused interests, becoming experts in their areas of passion.

Recognizing and nurturing these strengths can greatly benefit individuals with ASD, allowing them to excel in areas where their unique abilities shine. It also emphasizes the importance of providing opportunities that harness these strengths, promoting personal growth and success.

HOW DOES NEURODIVERSITY VIEW ASD?

Neurodiversity is a concept that recognizes and embraces the diversity of human brains and neurological differences. It emphasizes the idea that neurological variations, such as autism, ADHD, dyslexia, and others, are natural variations of the human brain rather than solely being seen as disorders that need to be cured or fixed. This concept promotes acceptance, understanding, and accommodation for individuals with different neurological makeups.

Neurodiversity views Autism Spectrum Disorder (ASD) as a natural variation in the human brain rather than solely as a disorder needing a cure or complete normalization. This perspective emphasizes several key points:

Diversity of Brains: Neurodiversity acknowledges that brains function differently across individuals. ASD represents a unique neurological wiring, which might present challenges in certain areas but can also bring forth exceptional abilities or perspectives.

Respect for Differences: It advocates for respecting and accepting these differences, considering them as part of the rich tapestry of human diversity. Rather than seeking to "fix" or eliminate these differences, neurodiversity encourages embracing and accommodating them.

Focus on Strengths: Instead of solely viewing ASD through deficits, neurodiversity highlights the strengths and positive aspects associated with it. Individuals with ASD often possess remarkable attention to detail, creativity, intense focus, and unique problem-solving skills.

Social and Environmental Factors: Neurodiversity recognizes that challenges faced by individuals with ASD often arise from societal expectations and environments that are not always conducive to their neurology. It aims to shift focus towards creating supportive environments and fostering acceptance rather than trying to make individuals conform to societal norms.

Advocacy for Inclusion: Neurodiversity advocates for inclusive practices in education, employment, and society. This means creating spaces and systems that accommodate diverse neurological needs, providing equal opportunities for success and participation.

Overall, the neurodiversity perspective challenges the traditional medical model that views conditions like ASD as inherently negative or in need of a cure. Instead, it promotes a more holistic understanding that values the diverse ways in which brains function

and contributes to creating a more inclusive and
accepting society.

CONCLUSION

Understanding autism spectrum disorder (ASD) is crucial in dispelling misconceptions and fostering a more inclusive society. In this book, we have meticulously tackled various misconceptions surrounding ASD. As we conclude this insightful journey, it's essential to emphasize the key takeaways and offer guidance on promoting a more accurate understanding of ASD.

One prevalent misconception is that ASD affects everyone in the same way. This book adeptly highlights the diversity within the spectrum, showcasing how individuals with ASD exhibit a wide range of strengths, challenges, and unique traits. This diversity requires a nuanced approach to support, acknowledging individual differences and strengths.

Another misconception often encountered is the belief that individuals with ASD lack empathy or emotions. However, this book adeptly challenges this by illustrating how people with ASD might express empathy differently, but their feelings are as genuine and deep as anyone else's. By emphasizing these emotional connections, this book contributes significantly to reshaping societal perceptions.

Furthermore, the exploration of the sensory experiences of individuals with ASD is enlightening. Many misconceptions arise from a lack of understanding regarding sensory sensitivities. This book illuminates how individuals with ASD can experience sensory information differently, underscoring the importance of creating sensory-friendly environments to accommodate these differences.

One of the most critical aspects addressed in this book is the misconception that ASD is a result of bad parenting or upbringing. By providing evidence-based insights, this harmful misconception is dismantled, highlighting that ASD is a neurodevelopmental condition with a strong genetic basis. This understanding helps reduce stigma and blame often unfairly directed toward families.

Moreover, emphasis on the strengths and talents of individuals with ASD contributes immensely to reshaping societal attitudes. By showcasing the unique abilities and contributions of individuals on the spectrum, this book champions a more inclusive narrative, fostering appreciation for diverse talents and perspectives.

Moving forward, it's crucial to continue advocating for awareness and acceptance. Education remains pivotal in reshaping societal attitudes toward ASD. Encouraging open dialogue, promoting acceptance, and advocating for inclusive policies are essential steps toward creating a world where individuals with ASD are fully embraced and supported.

This book stands as a testament to the power of education and empathy in challenging misconceptions and fostering a more inclusive society. It's a valuable resource that will undoubtedly contribute to a more compassionate and understanding world for individuals with ASD.

www.ingramcontent.com/pod-product-compliance
Lightning Source LLC
Chambersburg PA
CBHW050045260726
48658CB00005B/1781